BROKEN VESSEL

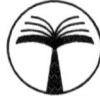

PALMETTO

PUBLISHING

Charleston, SC

www.PalmettoPublishing.com

Paperback ISBN: 979-8-8229-3097-1
eBook ISBN: 979-8-8229-3098-8

BROKEN VESSEL

Hidden Gems Found Through My Experience with Endometriosis Pain

ARIEL SPOERLE

DEDICATION

My husband, who has been my solid support and true friend. Thank you for all your help in my life.

My family and friends, who have blessed me in so many ways throughout the difficult years. I hope that I have loved you all well in return.

Women with endometriosis because you are brave to face each day. Your losses are many, but life is worth living.

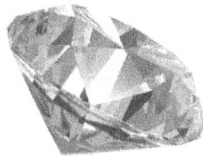

TABLE OF CONTENTS

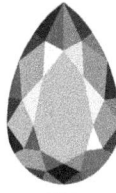

INTRODUCTION

I wrote this book for a few important reasons. In it, I explain my experience with endometriosis, and I hope that it will encourage others with endometriosis that they are not alone in their suffering and lived experience. I share what God has shown me at different times and how it changed my life for the better. I wrote this to remember when the pain was stronger and impacted my life a lot more so that when I interact with those who are in worse pain than I am in now, I can be compassionate and understanding—because I have been there too. I wrote this book based on my memories because I am experiencing less suffering in the present. I may need one or more surgeries in the future, so when times become difficult, I want to remember that it is nothing new and remember what God has shown me. I want to remember that He has not deserted me in the past, and He will not desert me in the present or in the future. I understand that while I have had a lot of loss and suffering, others with this chronic disease have suffered greater losses than my own. I care about you, and I hope that this book will be useful to you. I would like this book to reach those who have suffered from or are suffering with endometriosis, to raise awareness, and to present some of the realities that are experienced by those with this disease, as well as some of the impacts of endometriosis on everyone who loves those who suffer from it. I wrote this book to share the hidden gems that God has given me through my experience with endometriosis.

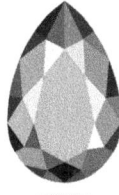

CHAPTER 1

Physical Pain
from Endometriosis

Today, I have pain less often, and it is not as wide-spread as it used to be because I received an excellent surgery. I do not think that I could write my story if I had the intense physical pain now that I had felt in the past, which was compounded by the tasks of life like work and chores. It took all my strength and deter-mination to give my best to my responsibilities, and I always fell short of my own desires because of the pain and exhaustion.

A couple of months before I turned thirteen, my periods started. I always had painful menstruation. After three years of experiencing pain during the days of menstruation, I started to feel pain every day of the month. I felt mild chronic pain in my pelvis and abdomen that would wrap around my low back for a couple of years. At the age of nineteen, the same constant pain had become a three to four level based on a scale from zero to ten. By the time I turned twenty-one, it had become a five to six level of pain, and I noticed that I was struggling more to get through each day. I started seeking medical care more often than I had attempted to in the past and still received no answers for a few more years. When I did receive the correct help, I had stage four endometriosis which is the most severe stage as far as I have been informed. Stage four is determined by the quantity of growths present and how deep they penetrate. Stage one consists of a smaller quantity of growths that penetrate less when compared to stage four of endometriosis. I was at a constant pain level of eight by the time I was diagnosed.

My pain increased through the years. I did feel an eight to ten level of pain for several years and had constant bleeding every day for one year before I received my first excision surgery for endometriosis. I felt well for three months after the surgery. After this, I was in eight-plus pain daily for two and a half years before receiving another excision surgery which brought me more freedom from pain for a long period of time. After the surgery, I was told that some endometriosis was left behind to preserve one of my organs for hormone balance until the time came when it would need to be removed later. This led to annual imaging and checkup appointments along with continuing to receive pelvic floor physical therapy. Endometriosis impacts your finances and time for sure!

I am going to describe the different types of pain that I experienced when the pain level was an eight and beyond so that others can understand them, and those who have this terrible disease can relate. I want endometriosis sufferers to understand that when I share the gems that benefited me and that I believe came from God, I was suffering. He is present. This is hard to fathom while living in such intense pain for so long. Please do not give up, do not end your life, and do not reject God, especially if you have already accepted Him into your life. Sharing about my pain will help me to remember it so that I can assist others who are experiencing intense pain from endometriosis.

The eight-plus pains were constant. I experienced deep pain that felt fiery and left a burning sensation. It was sharp, and at different times, it would be dull and achy instead. I had pains that would shoot up the sides of my body, and at other times, pains that would shoot down the insides of my legs. The pains in my pelvis always wrapped around my low back so my whole midsection hurt all the way around. There would be sudden moments when I had ten-plus pains that caused me to bend over. I would go to the emergency room for many of the ten-plus pains until I realized it was pointless because nothing they gave me would decrease my pain, not even morphine. When I took the hormones that a gynecologist prescribed to me for a few months, the pain went down from a constant eight to a constant six. I had severe side effects from taking the hormones after the first month, so I chose not to use that option after three months of trying it. I would get pains that felt like fists clenching me, but these locations never went numb, and these pains were some of the most unbearable for me. The constant eight-plus pains for days and years on end also disrupted my sleep, so I lived feeling constant fatigue. I tried to curl up in a ball for sleep, but many nights, I rolled or tossed side to back to side and never found a comfortable position. This disease literally exhausted me and impacted every part of my life. The pains made me cry a lot because of their intensity and their effect on me. I did not have the strength I once did, even when I had experienced milder chronic pain. I did not have the same thoughts or attitude as before because everything was so difficult. I did not have the life that I always dreamed I would have, and I did not have the strength to work toward my life goals. I felt that I had lost and was continuing to lose so much. I missed the healthy, well-rested, and less pain-filled me. The physical pain changed me at my core, which I will cover in the next chapters.

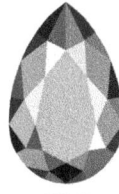

CHAPTER 2

Social and Emotional Pain from Endometriosis

If you're reading this right now, especially if you have endometriosis, I want you to know that you are not alone in your suffering. I know that you may not have close relationships with others because of your pain and that you fear losing any positive relationships that you do have. Please do not give up. Please know that you are important. I could never endure endometriosis without knowing Jesus as my God and Savior and having His Spirit dwelling in me. He is present. He is with you through every aspect and impact of it. I believe in heaven, and I believe that there is no sickness and death in it. I believe that God did not create sicknesses, and I trust that He will eliminate death once and for all in the future. Your illness, pain, and suffering were not designed by Him. Imperfect bodies that do not function in perfect health are part of living on a fallible earth. Perfection is not part of this time and existence, but I believe that people long for it because the time is coming when Jesus will return or when we meet Him before then and all will be renewed. I hope that you can place your hope in Jesus as your God and Savior and in the eternity that He has for everyone who receives Him.

God is relational, so I shared about Him and His help before explaining some of my experiences with social pain which causes emotional pain for me as well. People can withdraw from those who suffer from endometriosis for a few reasons. They do not understand your sickness and may not believe you when you describe your suffering. They are afraid to be close to you because of possibly losing you when you undergo surgeries or emergencies. They are more active, have healthier friends, and may choose not to make time to visit, assist, or listen to you. They may misunderstand your facial expressions and body language when you react to the constant pain as something negative directed at them, but you do not feel any ill will toward them at all. Some people may feel responsible for supporting you, but feel defeated when they give help, and it does not reduce your pain. People may be caring for one or more people already and cannot assist you too. People may be facing their own health struggles which prevents them from helping you or others. This is understandable since it is hard to assist others as much as you would like, or even at all, when you are facing endometriosis. People may not be ready to come alongside you or to be your friend while you battle endometriosis.

I have lived through and experienced not being able to attend small and large social functions multiple times throughout the years because of pain or heavy bleeding, and the invitations stopped being made because I was so often unable to go. I understand making the decision not to go to social events when you are exhausted from pain, feel short-tempered, and unable to interact in a socially acceptable manner. I can relate to feeling an inability to control your emotions in reaction to your pain, so you may choose to withdraw even from those you live with because you do not want to hurt them, and you are struggling to endure your pain. It is hard to live well when you feel like you are giving your all to survive. I felt a great struggle to maintain positive relationships while living in a high level of pain for an extended amount of time.

Social media contributed to both my social and emotional pain but was beneficial in some ways. I would see happy posts from friends about being pregnant, having and raising children, and I felt hurt that I was unable to enjoy their experiences because of my infertility. I felt depressed and jealous. Support groups on social media for women with endometriosis comforted me a little. I felt isolated from and not connected to friends on social media for several years until I accepted my inabilities and that I may not get everything that I want in life especially in the way or within the time that I desire. I may be older when I achieve my dreams or I may never do all that I want to accomplish, but life is still beautiful and worth living. There is still a purpose in my existence and a reason for my dreams. There is a beauty in accepting my life for how it is and not trying to force what I want to happen into existence. There is a beauty in letting go of expectations that I placed on myself and others and choosing to accept things for how they are. Lowering expectations and having a genuine acceptance for the present have been valuable things that I have learned. All the chores do not have to be done all the time. It is fine to ask for help with the chores. Things do not have to be done perfectly. Effort counts. Say, "Thank you," to those who assist you, those who care, those who listen, those who pray with and for you, and those who do your surgery, physical therapy, and so on. Thank God for the ability to live, to pray to Him, and to praise Him. Be grateful for anything you can, no matter how small.

Life may seem dark and empty to you. The walls of where you live may be so familiar to you that you feel trapped in them because of being in one place in pain for so long. I would be in bed, and my bedroom has white walls. I rent and am not allowed to paint them a different color, so I was sick of seeing the white walls in my room, at the emergency room, at the hospitals, and in gynecologists' offices. White walls were an unwanted and boring part of my existence, but I chose to be thankful that I had shelter at my apartment. I was not homeless. At the emergency rooms and hospitals that I went to, I was grateful that people were trying to help me. I tried to focus on and appreciate what I had instead of thinking about everything that I did not have.

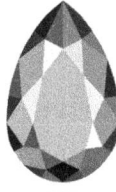

CHAPTER 3

Mental Pain from Endometriosis

In the last chapter, I discussed being thankful, and I have found the act of giving thanks very useful in overcoming the battle against negative thoughts. I struggled with making this chapter on mental pain separate from the chapter about social and emotional pain because I believe that all of them interconnect. The physical pain also connects to the other types of pain. This is my organization decision, so please feel free to see all the aspects intertwined, just like all the chapters make up this book. I am going to describe a few of the emotions that contributed to negative thoughts when I was in greater pain.

Depression was a part of my existence for a few years because of loss. I always wanted a large family, seven or more children, and to homeschool them, but I was infertile, and did not have the finances to adopt. I was devastated over my infertility and how it changed my whole life plan. I was sad about how slowly I could accomplish my goals in education. Around my pain, surgeries, and working a part-time job, it took me five years to earn two AA degrees. I did attend a few night and summer classes in person, but I took many classes online. It was easier on my strength levels to complete my classes from home instead of driving to and walking to classes on a campus. Pain would make it more difficult to think clearly and to work at a decent pace, but I maintained good grades, turned all my assignments in on time, and enjoyed keeping my mind active. I was able to perform well in my classes by choosing to take one to two classes per semester because this was the amount of schoolwork that I could do well around my other obligations in life. Some semesters, I would not enroll in classes if I had a surgery scheduled, and I was able to retain my qualification for financial aid. Praise from teachers on the work that I turned in was always encouraging. It felt good to be productive in the ways that I was able to during a time of physical weakness.

I think that boredom from rare occurrences of social interactions contribute to mental pain through self-doubt. Some of the thoughts that I had were, "I'm not healthy enough to have friends or visit with them or do activities with them, so they don't reach out to me," and "No one cares," and "No one believes me," and "I can't have friends without trust," and "No one listens," and so on. These were a few of the many hurtful thoughts that felt true because I was alone and in pain so often, without someone who could relate to me.

Fear was always an overpowering feeling that I had. Anxiety about what was causing so much pain before receiving a diagnosis. I was fearful when I did not know if I had cancer. The concern about cancer was further enforced later because I did have a gynecologist at one time do a blood test and state that cancer was a possibility. Worry about what was happening inside of me when I felt severe pain. Apprehension about whether my husband would remain faithful when I could not give him children and complete simple tasks at home. I felt concerned about my ability to maintain a job and about whether I could provide for myself because it was hard to show up and persevere through a part-time job on many days. Anxiety about the unknown, what answers may come later, and how they would impact my life. Worry about how the answers would impact my husband and those who loved me, who were in my life in small or big ways. Having the LORD, His peace, His Spirit, and His Word all helped, but I faced fear and sometimes experienced it or any of the other emotions and mental battles that I mentioned, for longer periods of time than I would have liked.

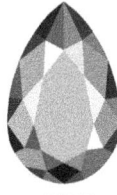

CHAPTER 4

Diagnosis

At the end of 2017, a gynecologist showed me my recent ultrasound images and discussed them with me. He stated that I had masses that appeared to be endometriomas, indicating that I had endometriosis. He explained endometriosis a little bit, handed me a brochure, and said that there was no cure. He also said that they determine whether it is endometriosis after doing a surgery. It is so defeating to be told that you have a disease that has no cure. After my diagnosis, I struggled with memories of people who had been unkind to me throughout the years that I had experienced pain. I wondered if they would be kinder to me now that I had a diagnosis that I could share to validate my previous and continuing symptoms and pain? In my battle with endometriosis, I have constantly felt that people do not believe me. Trust is vital to any relationship, so the pain of being distrusted goes deep. I had answers now, but I knew that if people had been inconsiderate so far, it was unlikely that they would treat me any better if I did share this information. I could not trust that unkind people would not try to hurt me more if I chose to share my diagnosis with them. The loneliness that you feel—even after a diagnosis supports you, your experience, and that you are honest, not crazy or making things up—is one of the hardest aspects of living with endometriosis.

In 2018, I had two surgeries for endometriosis and only a few months of decreased chronic pain after the second surgery which was done by excision. I had more relief and more ability to live life in an active and engaged manner after another surgery for the excision of endometriosis in 2021. It is the month of August in the year 2023, and I am writing this book to try to raise awareness and to be an encouragement to those who have experienced similar things if they are diagnosed with endometriosis. I know that this disease drains your finances, time, energy, and interrupts all parts of your life. This disease feels like a heavy burden and affects the lives of those who care about people with endometriosis too.

Before and after I received a diagnosis for endometriosis, having conversations with others about my experience was challenging. I dreaded conversations about endometriosis when they happened, and I still do if they are not with a person who has endometriosis, has had it, or has the skills and knowledge to assist those who are living with it. There were unhelpful statements that people made. One statement that I had heard a few times through the years was, "You look like you're fine." This statement hurt because the disease is inside you, so they cannot see it if they are not your surgeon or doing your medical imaging. There are many other illnesses that a person can face in life while looking fine on the outside. These illnesses can be invisible to others if they are inside you or in places under your clothing. I did not want to prove my sickness by lifting my shirt to show my scars from the surgeries that I had for endometriosis to be removed or show everyone who questioned my health the images that my surgeons had given me of the growths that had been in-side me at the time of surgery. Another upsetting state-ment that I heard was, "You must know how to handle pain well or be good at hiding it." This one caused pain because if you want to live in the outside world away from home so that you can make friends, go to work, or try activities, you must learn how to handle your pain. You are learning self-control, not how to hide pain, so the last part of the statement is a false accusation that is unsympathetic.

I think that a lot of people's hurtful statements come from their lack of knowledge about the disease and their inobservance. They do not know the subtle signs or do not care enough to take the time to observe or ask you about the symptoms of your pain. Some of my natural reactions to pain were resting my hand on the painful places like my abdomen or pelvis, tightening the muscles of my jaw, my pelvic floor muscles tight-ened because of the pain without any of my own added effort, and I would take deep breaths when I had sharp pain to prevent myself from screaming. I believe that my exhaustion was visible in the baggy and dark skin under my eyes. My ability to think and communicate became slower, and at times I was confused when I should not have been. When people say hurtful things, I think it is all right to share any truth that you feel the need to in a gentle and calm manner. If you do not feel the strength to give a calm response, you must learn to forgive and decide whether the person is a true friend and worth trying to keep in your life. If they are someone that you want to maintain a relationship with then you must arrange a time with them to discuss what you need to about their statement and how it affected you. This is challenging, and people do not always choose to trust you or remain in your life after these discussions.

I think it is important to be grateful for those in the healthcare profession who provide you care with physical therapy, surgery, and other parts of your experience while living with endometriosis. They care, they know the specific signs of your suffering, they have knowledge, and a willingness to help you. When others are letting you down or care but do not support you well then be more grateful for those who are assisting you. It is not necessary to explain your needs to others, unless you are trying to build a close bond with them, and they want to listen. This way, you can explain what you need to about how you react to or try to improve your pain, describe your suffering, and suggest how you could use their assistance. I think the best support oftentimes is having someone that is willing to listen and to help you with the tasks you cannot complete. Any person that is willing to listen to you, believe you, and support you, is someone that you should thank and recognize as a friend.

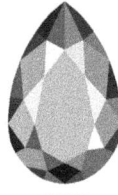

CHAPTER 5

Suffering and Scars

After I was told that I had endometriosis at the end of 2017, I was angry at God for a season that I remember lasting no longer than three months. I questioned why He would give me a deep desire in my heart during my growing-up years to have a family, and to be a mom, if He was going to prevent my ability to give birth naturally? I was poor financially, so adoption was not a possibility in the near future either. I did not understand God or my circumstances, so I became angry at Him. I did not want to seek His counsel or be close to Him. My pain was so deep that I chose to keep distant from Him.

I am grateful that He is a God who pursues, who is patient, who remains faithful, and who loves good and evil people. I am glad that He changes us for the better. My heart was hardened in that season of receiving the news about having an incurable disease. I was in severe chronic pain too, so I was in bed after work, on weekends, and on the holiday breaks from work, but after a few months God reached out to me.

One day, while I was lying in bed in physical agony, angry, and hurt emotionally, God spoke to me as that voice in the head that speaks to your heart and that you know is not yourself. He said, "Ariel, you're angry and hurt about being in bed from pain and about all the things that you can't do. Thank me for what you do have. Thank me for your salvation, your ability to make it to work, and pray to Me. By praying you are doing a lot. You can travel the whole world through praying from your bed." God provided healing for my deepest pain and acknowledged my deepest desire in these simple words. My heart softened, and I chose to obey Him. Many years after this experience, I have benefited from applying this wisdom. Many nights of disturbed sleep from pain would lead me to pray for others, relatives, friends, people I knew, and strangers. For believers and unbelievers. For those with endometriosis, other illnesses, and those living in places impacted by natural disasters, war, poverty, and so on. There is always someone to pray for somewhere.

I am crying as I write this because when I chose to obey God, He turned a dark, terrible, past, present, and ongoing experience in my life into something beautiful and powerful. There were many times when I felt so much pain and exhaustion that I was unable to think and pray. During these times, I trusted that Jesus was praying.

I have had a few surgeries for endometriosis, with at least one more expected in the future, but there could be more than that too. After my second surgery—not third, if I remember the timing correctly—I was struggling with looking at my scars. I was sad when I looked at my scars because they reminded me of all the pain, appointments, loneliness, and broken relationships that I had experienced. I do not know whether I questioned my beauty because of having them too, but if I did, it was in a small sense, and with the concern that my husband may think they were unattractive. The scars are under my clothing, so I did not question how they impacted my beauty too often because people were not looking at them. One day, while feeling sad as I looked at my scars in the mirror, that same voice in the mind happened again. God said, "Ariel, you're sad because your scars remind you of the pain that you have experienced. See them as proof of what I have brought you through." This touched me on a deep level again, and I did not struggle with looking at my scars when I applied the truth God had given to me. It takes remembering what He spoke and applying it for a while before it becomes natural and easier to do. God changed my mindset in these circumstances and gave me victory over them when I acknowledged His truth and obeyed His directions.

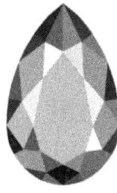

CHAPTER 6

Stronger and Sources That Encouraged Me

Some people think that the hardships in life make us stronger. I can understand that belief and I think it has some truth, but I do not consider it a full truth. I have words to express my feelings on the topic after living through many years without knowing how to respond to people when they said that I must be getting stronger through my experience with endometriosis. I am not strong in physical ways when my body is enduring a chronic and painful disease. The disease affects all parts of my life with pain, as I have written. There is strength in admitting that I am weak and entrusting God's Spirit to refine me as He wills. He has grown my self-control and perseverance. He has made me humble so that I seek Him for help. He has loved me and never left me in the suffering. He has been my strength. If you see strength in me, it is from God.

I have found and been given sources that have encouraged me throughout the years of pain. The Bible has been an encouragement to me most of my life especially after salvation. During my chronic pain within my years of marriage, my mother-in-law gave me a book that is one of my favorites, and I have shared it with others when they are facing troubling circumstances. It is called, *A Place of Healing: Wrestling with the Mysteries of Suffering, Pain, and God's Sovereignty*, by Joni Eareckson Tada. I told my mother-in-law that I liked Ellie Holcomb's songs, and she gave me a CD by her as a gift before I had to travel to some appointments. I enjoyed listening to the songs when traveling to appointments for endometriosis. My sister had a copy of the book, *Captivating: Unveiling the Mystery of a Woman's Soul*, by John and Stasi Eldredge, that she does not remember owning or giving to me, but I thought she did, so maybe I accidentally ended up with it when I moved away from home. I read this book a few times and it made me feel refreshed every time. I purchased the next couple of books by Ruth Chou Simons, and they encouraged me: *Beholding and Becoming: The Art of Everyday Worship*, and *When Strivings Cease: Replacing the Gospel of Self-Improvement with the Gospel of Life-Transforming Grace*. During a phone call with my maternal grandparents, they recommended this book, *The Priestly Prayer of the Blessing: The Ancient Secret of the Only Prayer in the Bible Written by God Himself*, by Warren M. Marcus, and I liked it. I have enjoyed Michael Card's music from a young age and up to the present. I love his book, *Inexpressible: Hesed and the Mystery of God's Lovingkindness*. One day, I was shopping with my mom at a little bookstore in Lake Arrowhead called Heart's Desire, and I found the following book, *Facing Illness with Hope: Leaning on Jesus*, which encouraged me a lot. When I was first told that I had endometriosis, I started doing research and found the *Endo What?* documentary, which was useful. I highly recommend it. Songs have and still do encourage me in my Christian faith and life circumstances. A few of my favorite music artists have been and are to this day: Toby Mac, Jason Gray, and Ellie Holcomb.

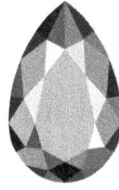

Giving My Thanks

I am thankful to God for rescuing me from my sin at a young age and giving me His Spirit so that I can live in His righteousness. I am grateful for His presence. I love because He loves me. I can give my thanks to others because of His love.

I am thankful for my husband, who has remained faithful through the pain, emergency room visits, surgeries, and recoveries, all these years. Thank you for assisting me with daily tasks and holding me through many tear-filled hours during the pain I was experiencing.

Thank you, relatives, and friends, for supporting me during recoveries from surgeries in the ways that you were able to. My mom, stepdad, and grandparents visited me at the hospital for a couple of my surgeries. My sister, brother-in-law, and niece visited me at the hotel that I was in after my third surgery. My family's presence encouraged and comforted me during those difficult times. My in-laws provided resources of encouragement and support. Sierra Robinson spent a week or longer assisting in the care I needed during a recovery from one of my surgeries for endometriosis. Her help relieved my husband of some of the work of taking care of me, and her presence in the same place as us was good for our emotional well-being. Sierra's presence prevented us from feeling alone in the recovery process which was a need that we had. Thank you, relatives and friends who prayed.

I am grateful for everyone who came alongside me throughout the years. Thank you to those who listened to me. Thank you to those who gave resources, hugs, physical labor, finances, emails, texts, and mailed cards that had Bible verses and handwritten words of encouragement. There are many names that come to mind, but I want to respect privacy. Please know that if you were someone who helped me even once, even if you have been kind to me without any knowledge about my struggles, that I appreciate you. I am grateful to those who were understanding, kind, and supportive.

Thank you to all the healthcare workers and professionals who have worked with me through the years and those that still are. Your knowledge and love shown to your patients do not go unnoticed. I have a special appreciation for the physical therapists that I have had.

Thank you to all my college professors for all that you taught me. Thanks to you, I grew in my knowledge and understanding of life. I am thankful for each of you who provided positive feedback on my assignments. Thank you to those who were mentors and teachers to me outside of the classroom and college setting, people at work, friends in their homes, and those who reached me with encouragement without even knowing it through their written works.

People who could make me laugh during the hard times blessed me more than they know. I am grateful for some people that I have never had the pleasure of meeting.

Thank you to those who assisted me with the publishing process and everyone who purchases my book.

I hope that my thankfulness can be contagious and motivate those who have endometriosis to give thanks for one or more people in their lives and sphere of influence. Giving thanks will be beneficial to you and to those you show appreciation to. Everyone that I thanked and everyone who helps people with chronic illnesses, as well as God's messages to me, are hidden gems that I found in my experience with endometriosis.

Sincerely,

Ariel Spoerle

REFERENCES

Card, Michael J. 2018. *Inexpressible: Hesed and the Mystery of God's Lovingkindness*. Westmont, IL: IVP Books.

Cohn, Shannon, et al. 2016. *Endo What?* Endo What.

Eldredge, John, and Stasi Eldredge. 2010. *Captivating: Unveiling the Mystery of a Woman's Soul*. Nashville, TN: Thomas Nelson.

Marcus, Warren M. 2018. *The Priestly Prayer of the Blessing: The Ancient Secret of the Only Prayer in the Bible Written by God Himself*. Lake Mary, FL: Charisma House.

Simons, Ruth Chou. 2019. *Beholding and Becoming: The Art of Everyday Worship*. Eugene, OR: Harvest House Publishers.

———. 2021. *When Strivings Cease: Replacing the Gospel of Self-Improvement with the Gospel of Life-Transforming Grace.* Nashville, TN: Nelson Books.

Tada, Joni Eareckson. 2010. *A Place of Healing: Wrestling with the Mysteries of Suffering, Pain, and God's Sovereignty.* First ed. Colorado Springs, CO: David C. Cook.

Wesemann, Rev. Tim. 2009. *Facing Illness with Hope: Leaning on Jesus.* Fenton, MO: CTA.

Milton Keynes UK
Ingram Content Group UK Ltd.
UKHW020637110124
435856UK00016B/413

9 798822 930971